# WAKE UP AND WORKOUT 2nd edition

## HOW I LOST NEARLY 100 LBS IN 1 YEAR

By Deidra Jones

# WAKE UP AND WORKOUT

## Table of Contents

# PREFACE

Too often we find ourselves in a daily rut, not realizing the changes going on around us, and sometimes within us. When awareness to the behavior that causes our malfunctions arise, we make excuses to justify why we have not corrected our behavior, in some cases, falsely blaming others for our lifelong failures. We continuously go through life, making the same mistaken choices over, and over. Excusing others' shortcomings as if we are excusing our own, creating a society of incorrect behavior, eventually passing those unhealthy habits on to our offspring. Leaving us to later wonder, "what happened to the world?" How can we ask that question, without first looking at ourselves? But it can't be me...right? ...right.

If I interact with the world, I, in some way, will influence the world. The effect may be minute, but it is still an effect, an effect that could spread. I have concluded that, that is the reason we have realized change begins with self. How can we expect the world to change if we ourselves cannot commit to the task? Why do we expect change in the world, while we stay the same? Continuing the same behavior, expecting different results is the definition of insanity. We are insane! There is ugliness in the world this is also in us. We know we have it yet do nothing to change the ugliness. We know we are not healthy but will not do anything to change that. Our eyes keep looking out over the horizon for someone else to do something, while ignoring our own responsibilities. No one is going to come show you how to cook a healthy meal or tell you that you need to work out. No one is going to get you into that mindset except for you. The will to want change is in you. The want to have change is in you. The power is in you.

Losing weight and staying healthy is not just about the way you look it is also about the way you feel. There is nothing better than feeling light and energized. Of course, we want those clothes to fit nice too. There is a misunderstanding that if you are not fat, you are healthy. That is not true. However, being overweight can be a sign of being unhealthy, but so can being underweight. Looks can be deceiving, so weight is not the only telling factor. What is your energy level like? What are your cholesterol levels? Do you have headaches and body aches? Are you a diabetic? Have high blood pressure? Can you bend over and touch your toes? Sometimes it is just the trivial things, the things that we cannot see that are symptoms of poor health.

We do not see being healthy as being responsible, we see it as a chore that we only needed occasionally, instead of viewing it as a lifestyle. I thought keeping my weight in check with a healthy diet and exercise was only necessary if I were to get "too big." Ignoring the fact that a healthy diet and exercise is what I needed to keep me from getting "too big." As an adult I did not realize that fast food was a "sometimes food" as a child for a reason. Bedtime was for a reason. My being allowed to rarely eat sweets, was for a reason. "You can do what you want to do once you are grown" is the worst thing to tell a child. You most certainly cannot! Once you stray from what is right, you will surely stroll down the path of wrong.

As you can tell, I have learned my lesson and have decided to get myself right...body, mind, and spirit. The spirit had to be the first to get into gear because it controls the mind and body. I had to remove all negativity about my plan to achieve my goal, leaving only room for positivity. My positivity had to speak louder to me than the distractions and negative people in my life.

You may even have to put one or two relationships on hold until you have achieved your goal. (Sometimes, the bulk of the weight you will lose, is from "Negative Nellies.") My want for results had to be stronger than my want for some junk food or to want to lounge instead of working out. Using my spare time wisely for "me time," became a priority. And knowing what "me time" and "self-care" really means is necessary. My mindset about what I put into my body had to change. I had to change. With those changes came a lot less of being tired, which triggered unnecessary anger. You would be surprised at what less anger in your life would do for relieving stress. Relieving stress will alleviate headaches, and with less pain, again less anger...better life.

Nothing in this book says, "easy." Nothing in life worth doing is easy. Your will and desire must be strong enough...you must care. Sometimes we need trick the mind with games and rewards, whatever it takes to get to your goal. But even the tricks are proof of your desire for change. You should handle tricks and rewards like training wheels; you use them at the beginning, but you will not need them forever. We usually crawl before we walk, so do not rush the change, but keep pushing yourself to get to the next level.

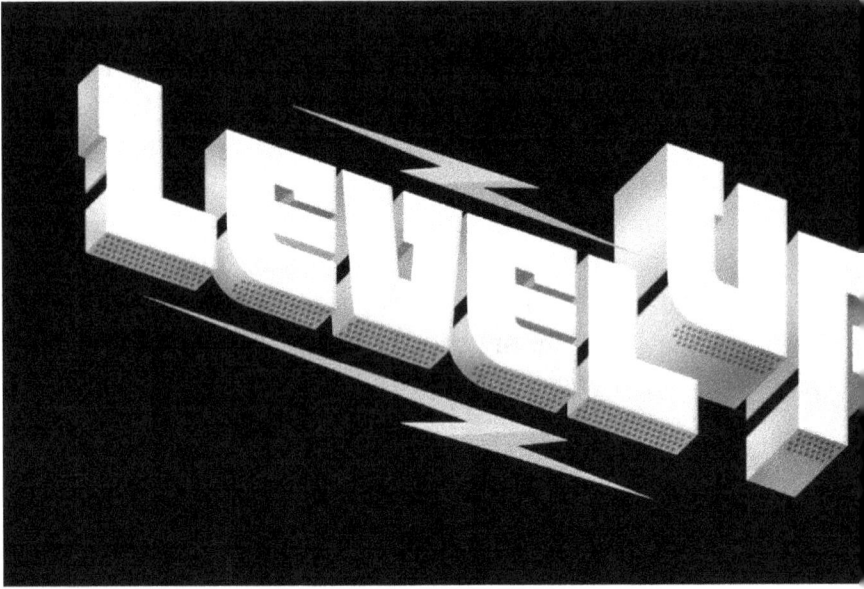

Being a single mother of two, I did not pay attention to my weight, I am embarrassed to say I did not really pay attention to my looks altogether. There was not enough time between my career and my children. At least that is how it seemed. I honestly did not have time to try and impress anyone (especially a mate). There was no time for me, so there is surely no time for anyone else. Mom always said that if you are clean and neat, the rest is irrelevant.

So, I made those words my motto not realizing that I was ignoring the most important matter, my health. In these times, when viruses are morbid simply because of underlying health problems, ignoring my health could be deadly. My focus was not on the root of my problem. I was neat and clean on the outside, the inside I was not. I was proud of myself for making a mess look quasi-presentable.

The sad thing about life is, I still had to look at myself in the mirror daily. That mirror can be a vicious creature! It is there, mocking you, making you look at yourself in disgust every day. You ignore the signs of being unhealthy, so you continue to be lazy, drowning out any words of encouragement from T.V. and social media ads to workout, eat right, and lose weight. Who wants to trade the wonderful thing they have going for exercise? Who wants to ditch their favorite comfort food for a healthier choice? There is a saying, "The truth hurts..." The mirror gives it to you, the cold hard truth, and it does not care if you like it or not. It gives you the truth day in and day out.

You either ignore the signs in the mirror or change your view. And when I say change your view, I do not mean for you to look elsewhere. I mean change what your mirror reflects at you. I have ignored that mirror for a long time. It is time to change my view!

For a lot of us, change is not easy at all. For some, they just need a little time to adjust. And for others change is a breeze. If you fight against the change, you just make things harder for yourself. Pick your battles. You want to become victorious with the least amount of resistance as possible. Besides, we already have enough on our plates, there is no need to add hurdles.

When I say change, what do I mean? Let us start with a definition or two:

1a: to make different in some way

2 b: to make radically different

c: to give a different position, course, or direction to

3a: to replace with another

b: to make a shift from one to another

c: to exchange for an equivalent sum of money (as in smaller denominations or in a foreign currency)

Living a certain way for several years, is not going to change with a snap of the fingers. Like a vehicle with momentum, your lifestyle will not just stop and change direction instantly. Change takes time... at least any change that is going to stick with you, takes time. However, you must be persistent, you cannot be lackadaisical in your efforts.

What does change begin with? We say that change begins with you. OK. Now that we have got that out of the way. What does that mean? Well... what makes you, you? I am going to say, how you think and act, or your personality is what makes you who you are. What type of person are you? Lazy? Focused? Practical? Logical? How do you receive and apply information? Are you open to learning information new to you? Will you learn something new and apply it right away? Or will you learn something new and fight with adjusting to your new findings? Depending on your answers to those questions, there may be some room for change. Although it is necessary, change is never easy, but that depends on your personality.

I believe the largest part of the struggle of losing weight and staying healthy, is the mental struggle. That little voice can be so negative at times, always yelling what you cannot do, instead of telling you what you can. If you say you cannot do something, you will believe you cannot. If you believe you cannot do something, then you will not. The mind controls the brain, which controls the body. The stronger the mind, the stronger the body can become. The most popular song you would hear me sing was, "I don't feel like...." So, of course, I did not feel like... I was unconsciously allowing my brain, to tell my body, not to want to do anything. There is no room for negativity. Negativity can be the biggest downfall towards any progress or success. As soon as I said, "I don't feel like...", guess what? I do not feel like.... The first thought of, "I can't" replace it with action (I can). In other words, if you feel yourself saying or about to say, "I can't", begin replacing inaction with action. Immediately move towards and begin the task at hand. Once you begin, you will forget you did not want to start. Try it and watch the results!

My daily routine was to get up and get ready for work (which got harder to do each day). I produced and directed my children's daily routine before taking them to their destination. After fighting traffic for over an hour, I would sit on my butt for eight hours or more at work. We all know jobs that allow you to sit all day are not healthy, add stress to that and you have yourself a big pot of "Underlying Condition" soup. After a day of sit-n-stress, it is time to pick up my children and fight traffic for over an hour and a half to get home. Time for rest?... nope! Dinner needs be prepared and the kitchen cleaned up afterwards. And please do not let there be a bunch of homework! Wind down for a few, and then off to bed and repeat.

One day, while going through my daily routine, putting on my clothes, I noticed they were fighting back and fitting a bit tight. At first, I thought I may have shrunk my clothes in the wash. But every day, each outfit was getting tighter and tighter. Even the material that was supposed to stretch stopped stretching. I also my constant fatigue and I would breathless be breathless walking up the stairs to my front door. At age 30 or any of the 30's, you should not have a problem taking on the same 15 stairs you climb daily.

I noticed I would sweat profusely, even when the weather was cool. After showering, sweat would keep pouring, causing me to want to shower again. You would think it was the steam, but the moisture would continue to stream well after I had gotten dressed. I had no energy and never wanted to take part in any activities that involved leaving the house. To give you an idea of how little energy I had, my kids did not mind teaming up with me on Call of Duty. That is a video game for those that do not know. And that is how well I played the game.

Concerned I might have some type of health condition, I made an appointment to see my doctor. After expressing my concerns about my symptoms, I waited to hear the worst. I just knew the doctor would relay that I have some awful condition or sickness that I would need surgery for or would have to take medication for the rest of my life. After hearing so many health horror stories over the years, I did not know what to expect, I just knew it would not be good.

My doctor is very professional and tried to still be so as she tried to hold her amusement at my concerns. She looked at the monitor for a small pause. I could tell she did not want to hurt my feelings when she broke it to me... "Before we look into any health problems, we have to first discuss your weight." OK... dagger!

I was a bit overweight... Ok I was very overweight. For my body frame and height, I am supposed to weigh 130 lbs-135 lbs. I weighed in at a whopping 198 lbs.! How could you not notice you have gained a half of a person that you are toting around? I was embarrassed at this point. I came into the doctor's office crying about illnesses and medication, when all I need is a better diet, and some exercise. I know I am not alone, and some, if not all of you know how I am feeling. LOL! I thought I was going to be doing something as simple as popping a pill or two. The true remedy was putting in some work. I must take responsibility for myself. At this point having self accountability is the realization that I have been avoiding and deflecting for far too long.

*"The first step, is admitting there is a problem"*

From the time that we are children until adults, if not from our parents, in school, and even through movies and television to, "eat right and exercise!" But do we listen? No. We go about life, behaving as if our childhood bodies will remain the same highly energized, healthy vessel it has been since birth with no effort to help it remain that way. How delusional could we be? Especially if you have children. There is no way we are going to still be a size 2 all our lives (I will make note of the exceptional few out there). I thought I could remain petite... didn't you? Lol!

I ignored the fact that my clothes kept getting tighter and tighter, the low energy, and the fatigue. I just chalked it up to my clothes shrinking in the wash. Now, what do you do when your clothes shrink in the wash? You go buy more of course! Well, this is where my life, the one I was living in my head, and reality merged. "Are they using funhouse mirrors in the fitting rooms?" "These clothes have the wrong sizes tagged on them." "I guess the sizes are made smaller now." Those were my thoughts while having to do something I absolutely despise. I absolutely loathe shopping for clothes and now add into the mix that I must now buy bigger sizes?!...damn!

Nothing fits right. Nothing looks right. The styles I liked seemed cute, but only in smaller sizes. The larger dresses and tops seemed like 2 large pieces of material, sewed upon the sides to close the garment, leaving an opening on each side for arms, and a hole at the top for a head to go through. No shape in the material to reflect it was for a woman's body. Sometimes the larger sizes did not even resemble the smaller size. Hey designers, what is up with that? Even though a woman may be a bit overweight, she would still like to show her femininity. ...I digress, unhappy with shopping, I just did not buy any clothes for a while. But now I am stuck with clothes that do not fit. It is either clothes that do not fit, or the frumpy look. Decisions, decisions... Do not misunderstand me, there are some women that make those larger sizes work. I am just not one of them.

So now what? Should I never go anywhere because I have nothing to wear? I have children, a job, and somewhat of a life, I cannot do that! Not to mention, that does not make any sense at all. Should I continue to ignore my looks, and be angry when I look at myself in the mirror? No way! That is just a road to depression highway. I love myself too much for that, and I have never been a quitter. I always tell myself, and others that need to hear it, "If you do not like something about yourself, change it!" Change is what I intend to do!

# THE FIRST STEP

The first step is noticing there is a problem. If you do not ever see anything wrong with yourself, you will not see a need to make changes or to do better for yourself. We tend to make idle excuses when we do not believe, or do not want to believe anything is wrong with ourselves. The kind of excuses like the one I used about my clothes shrinking in the wash. The most common excuse is, "I don't have enough time." To me, excuses are a form of procrastination. When you take the time to sit down and really breakdown the excuses, they are just a hindrance to progress. They are illusions we put up, so others will not know that we are truly lazy, enjoy, and do not want to change our current situation whether it ruins our health or not. We look at others with similar lifestyles and look at them thinking they look ok, so what I am doing is fine. Looks can be deceiving. They may look well, but are they well? Could there be some major illness building up that you and that person have no clue is to soon manifest? Does that person know they are unhealthy, but wants you to continue to believe they are healthy? People lie to themselves as well as others all the time. (There is that hurtful truth again.). Excuses and procrastination never got anything done.

Remember when you were a child? You felt like the days were long, and life would never end. You believed you had all the time in the world to change the world if you even pondered time at all. School kept you active, and social life kept you distracted. No thought about exercise and diet. At least that is my story.

Life moves fast once you leave school. As time flies by, we forget to pay attention to how we change along with our lives. Next thing you know, we are adults... we have changed. Our routine has changed. Our belief has changed. Our body has changed. While trying to survive, or what is commonly known as "living," it never comes to mind to watch for a metabolism shift as you get older so that you may adjust your diet. Or start a workout regimen because you notice you are not as active as you used to be when you were in school. Family comes along, and your primary concern is their health. Your family's wellbeing is priority over your own, so you sacrifice yourself into work to earn enough for their nourishment and shelter. You make a fuss over foods and the snacks they eat. You make sure they make it to their doctor and dental appointments while missing your own. Your family is healthy, but what about you? If you were no longer there, where would your family be? To take care of others, you must make sure you are able. Which means you must take care of self-first. It may sound selfish but could not be more selfless. A family is a tree of branches which stem from a trunk, and that trunk formatted at the root. If the root is weak or dead, the branches will not survive.

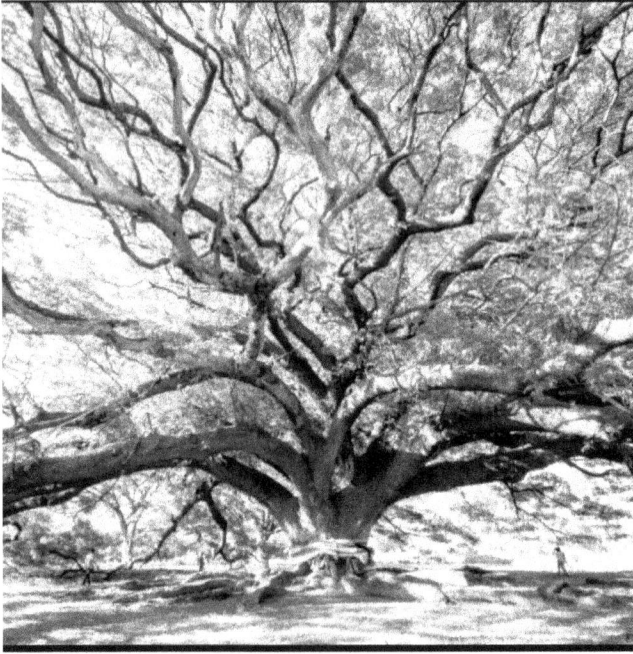

No one is talking about how you have gained weight... at least not in your face. I have learned, you cannot always depend on friends and family to tell you you have gained weight, or that you are not looking healthy. Some fear you may get angry, others fear you might point out their lil extra weight or imperfections. So, to them, you always look good. Your significant other may just not want to start an argument or make you feel insecure, so they may act as if nothing is wrong.

You must be real with yourself. You know whether you are living healthy. If you do not know, consult a health professional, which you should do regularly anyway. There are some things you do not need a doctor to tell you is wrong. One of the identifiers of something being wrong, is being overweight. Headaches for no reason is another. Fatigue and low energy are a couple more symptoms of something being wrong. We should not wait until these problems affect us, but once we do, we want to run to the doctor looking for medication and surgeries.

Do you drink alcohol? Put it down. Do you drink soda/pop? Pour it out. Do you eat sweets? Toss 'em. Are you aware that those things cause health problems? Especially with the preservatives and dyes that are in them known to cause health issues. If not, let me be the first to tell you, they cause health problems. Then you can let your doctor be the next to tell you. Those few things are not even scratching the surface of the harmful things we put in our bodies, but it is a place to start looking. I have never really eaten a lot of sweets. I did indulge, but not a lot. I was a huge fan of soda at one point in my life. That carbonated delight is addictive! I may have loved the taste, but it was destroying my body. When I learned the amount of processed sugar that was in soda, I dropped that habit quickly. The horror stories I had heard about diabetes were incentive enough to leave soda alone. Not everyone will stop cold turkey the way I stopped the soda because they are busy giving excuses. Other than giving excuses another strategy used, is ignoring, or downplaying the seriousness of a problem. The point is the excuses will not do anything to make your health better. I can either stop with the excuses or allow processed sugar, toxic dyes, and preservatives to continue to eat away at my body. Excusing away a problem has never proved successful. Once you ready to take accountability for yourself, with and stop fighting with yourself, gravity, health problems, and fatigue, you might finally be tired enough to do something about it.

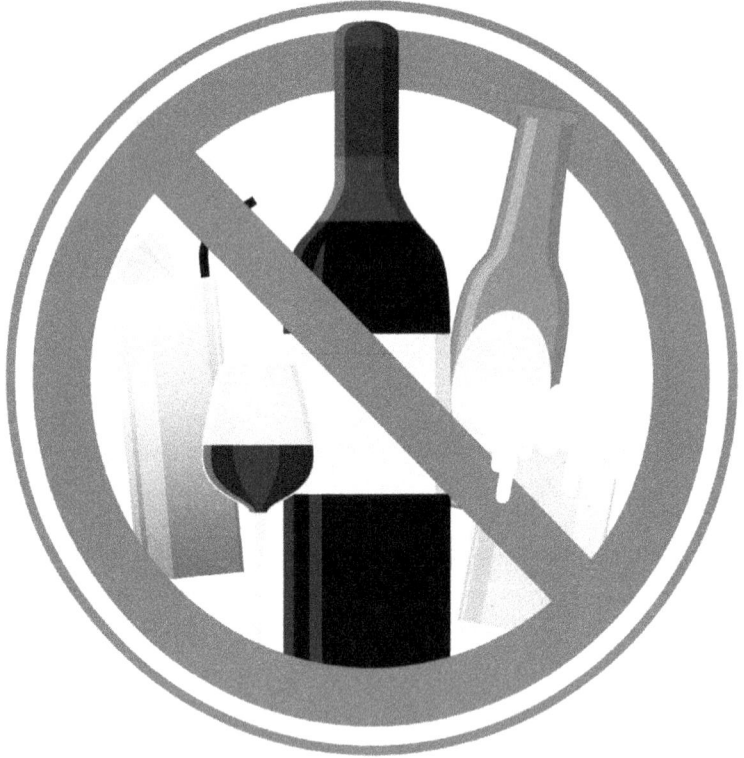

# UNDERSTANDING WHAT YOUR BODY NEEDS

Usually, if you are overweight, or even underweight, your body is starving for something it needs or dying from what it is getting. Of course, what we eat is important. What we put inside our bodies, reflect on the outside of our bodies. Staying away from processed or fake foods, incorporating more fresh fruits and vegetables in your diet, along with less meats and carbohydrates will help you reach your goal quicker. At least that is what worked for me. I used to believe it would be ideal for everyone to have the same plant-based diet. Plant-based diet does not mean meatless. It just means more fruits and vegetables in your diet, than meat. Men need meat more than women. To some of us, little to no meat on the plate is blasphemy. I used to believe every meal had to have some type of meat. With a little effort and research, I found that eating meat with every meal is unnecessary. We do not need meat, we want meat. I assume the desire for meat only exists because when you were a child you ate meat daily. If you never thought animals were edible, you would not eat rotting carcass. First, if grocery stores were not easily accessible, how many of us are going to slay an animal with our bare hands? And then to bleed and clean it before cooking is another task. Not me! If we had a worse case scenario, I might have to suck it up and return an animal back to the creator. But I will gladly plant and harvest fruits and vegetables. Fruits, vegetables, and legumes give the body everything thing it needs. Meat is extra.

Items you find super tasty, quick to grab, and easy to eat, are usually empty. They have no nutritional value, and they deceive you into thinking your body is satisfied. You can eat a ton of it and feel full, but your body is still starving. The body is a natural vessel, so it is only right to nourish the body with the things that nature provides us, that ensures the body will run at best performance.

I used to believe the easiest, cheapest choice to feed a family, was the dollar menu at the fast-food restaurants. There is not one nutritional item on any of the dollar menus out there. Which is why most will say it is more expensive to eat healthy than to not eat healthy. If we are being honest here, that is not a fact. Spending less to buy more of something unhealthy, is causing you to risk your health which is a bigger expense than a few more dollars. The health issues fast food can give will cause you to spend more on remedies such as medication or some type of medical attention. May cause an illness that will cause you to miss or even quit working. I believe fasting would be a better choice than filling your body with toxic foods. Also, you must pick up fast food daily, right? Why not fresh fruits and vegetables daily?... convenience. You do not have to get out of your car and walk to get fast food. You will not have to stand over a stove after working all day. Sometimes we must sacrifice convenience for our health. I am not saying you cannot go out for a meal occasionally. But do your research and make sure the food is clean and healthy, never fast. Fast food means something necessary for your food was omit or compromised.

 Your body needs plenty of water. One of my favorite sayings is, "Water is life." Hydrate your insides, as well as your skin (skin is an organ, it needs attention too). Water helps us to flush out the toxins in our bodies, keeps our body temperature regulated through urinating and sweating. The digestive system needs water to work properly to avoid constipation. Water delivers oxygen throughout the body via the blood, which helps the body convert what we eat into energy (metabolism).

Every morning, before eating or drinking anything, the first thing I would do, is drink a cup of warm water with a squeeze of lime. This helped with starting up the metabolism, and digestion

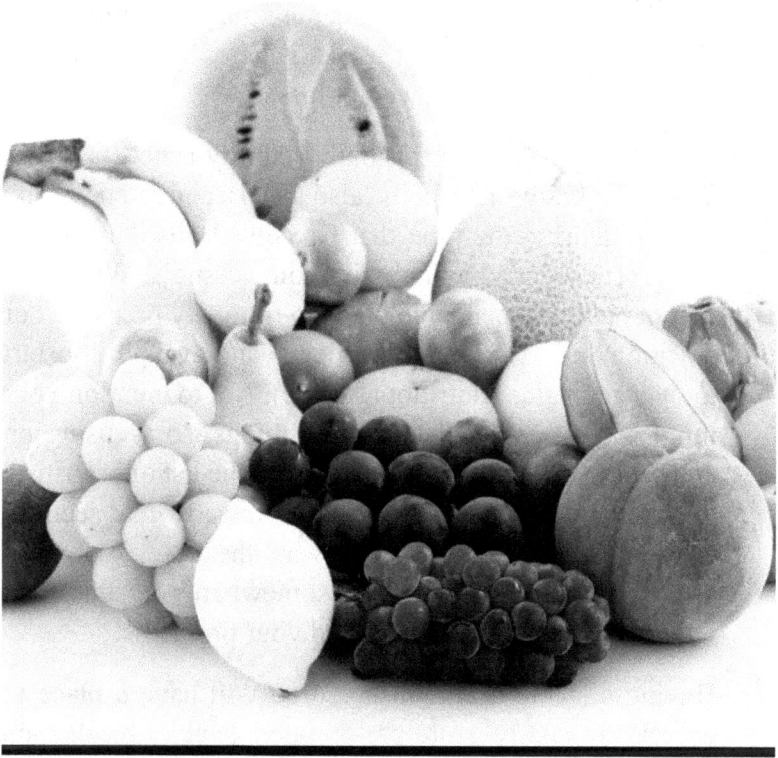

Later, I found out that ginger is a great digestion tool, so then I started my mornings steeping ginger root in water, also known as ginger tea. This helps with reducing bloating and helps with weight loss.

Although it may seem off-topic, stability is necessary for a healthy body. The body also needs consistency, and routine. During the time that I received this epiphany, I had recently ended a bout with homelessness. When you do not have a dependable place to routinely prepare your nutrition and exercise, convenience and availability start to override value (nutritional value). Not to mention your mind is pre-occupied with other things, so focusing on nourishment is not likely at the top of the list of priorities. It is understandable that you have concerns that seem to outweigh your health. However, the effort to keep yourself healthy should be somewhere on that list. Otherwise, you could compound your problems.

Having a stable home, insures you will have a place to exercise regularly, store pre-prepped, healthy meals, and boil water if times get too hard, or bottled water gets too expensive. Growing some of your own food would be ideal. Growing your own food allows you to keep a regular meal schedule and having a place to ensure proper rest. Instability brings clutter to your mind and your life. With clutter there can be no steady flow of energy. Without a steady flow on track, it will be difficult to still be on track.

Unbelievably, getting the proper amount of rest weighs in on how you keep your weight. While sleeping your body is processing the data it took in for the day. Necessary nutrients flow to their designated body parts. Unnecessary waist is prepared for disposal. So, everything your body took in that day will be the same things your body processes that night. How our bodies feel when we rise depend on what we did to and with our bodies the day before. I need at least 5 to 6 hours of sleep, to function properly the next day. If I sleep less than that, I am grumpy, looking for comfort foods which usually end up being something not so good for me. The reason for that is because I interrupted the processing of the nutrients, so I feel as if I had not eaten. I also noticed that when I stay up those extra hours, I eat extra snacks.

Having a set dinner time is helpful. I usually try to have dinner in between 4pm and 7pm. That way I have at least a few hours to digest my food before bedtime. If I get the urge to snack before bedtime I would have a light snack. For example, I would have a hand full of tortilla chips and salsa, a hand full of unsalted roasted peanuts, or lightly salted popcorn. Eating a meal too close to bedtime can cause trouble sleeping, heartburn, and weight gain. I learned that the hard way. The routine of having meals around the same time of day every day, helps with digestion. The body likes routine, and it has its own clock. Keep your body on a routine and in turn it will show appreciation by running like a well-oiled machine. Pre-planning and pre-prepping meals for the week not only helps you stay conscious of what you put into your body and when you put it in your body but can also help with budgeting and saving money. From time to time, we are hungry, short on time and money. That is when the dollar menu starts calling your name. Or the chips in the gas station seem to be a quick fix. But you are truly not fixing anything, you are starving your body. So, having something ready and waiting when that hunger strikes will be beneficial to your body, and to your finances.

Meal ideas and healthy preparation are things I had to gradually learn. The trick was to learn to prepare them in a way that I would still want to continue eating healthy. Because now the goal is to prepare meals with less salt, processed sugar, and fat. My goal was to eventually cut meat and dairy from my diet, but gradually so. My reason for wanting to cut out eating chicken was because I would get headaches after eating any chicken dish. Beef made me feel sluggish after consumption. And dairy, if made with cow's milk, is horrible on my digestive system. When I first authored this book (this is a revision of the original) I was not wise to the fact that it was not just the meat but what was in the meat that was causing my issues. The problem was the same with dairy. There were chemicals in the meats and dairy that my body did not agree with. I had the opportunity to eat meat outside of the United States and had none of the symptoms I have incurred from eating meat at home. So, with that said I believe that if we are going to consume meat it should be clean.

Since I was not the world's worst when it came to preparing meals, it was the horrible snacking habit I tackled first. I love potato chips, corn chips, tortilla chips, cheese puffs, anything with a crunch and some flavor. And of course, there is the dip. Naturally, certain chips we must dress with dip. Sometimes the dip was a processed cheese. Not particularly good altogether. Let us not forget my childhood bestie, milk chocolate. Oh yes, and donuts! Those were all my comfort foods. Not easy giving up the comfort foods, especially when you are going through challenging times.

Non-nutritious snacking is a not so good habit (even when you are going through tough times). To get rid of the bad habit, we replace it with a good habit. We never get rid of "bad" habits; we just replace them. But how do we carry out this feat? And with what? Well, someone must have heard my cry, because I just so happened to come across this recipe called "Cowboy Caviar." (Recipes in the back of the book) Made with black beans and other fruits and veggies that are nutritious. You still use tortilla chips to scoop and eat the salad, you just do not use Doritos. You can, but not if you want to lose weight. You may want to find some lightly salted or unsalted tortilla chips. I like the ones lightly salted with the lime salt. You can have Cowboy Caviar as a meal, lunch, or dinner. I also found kale chips to be a great snack. Especially if you just have the munchies (want to snack, but not hungry). Kale chips are an all-natural, tasty snack even your pickiest child would love! Of course, you can never go wrong with snacking on fresh fruits and vegetables when you have a sweet tooth.

You could have called me the queen of sandwiches back in the day (peanut butter and jelly being my favorite) until I realized bread went against the very thing I was trying to do. And since I enjoy peanut butter and jelly sandwiches immensely, I found a way to enjoy the taste, without the bread. At first, I used to spread peanut butter on Ritz crackers and top them with either blueberries or raspberries, or both. Sometimes with strawberries, other times with apples. I later realized those crackers, as tasty as they are, were not helping my cause. So, I learned to mix peanuts and blueberries and or raspberries in a bowl. And sometimes I would mix in a little vanilla flavored granola…delicious!

Another healthy snack that is easy to keep on you always are roasted almonds. They seem to keep you satisfied until the next meal. I would not select any candied or salted options. Go for the roasted, unsalted choice. Even give the dark chocolate covered version a try. They are quite filling, you only need a few, and they do not taste bad.

I used to like to drink soda/pop a lot when I was a child. In my adult years, it became something to drink with a meal. I found that all soda/pop and juices with high fructose corn syrup and unnatural sugars were detrimental to losing weight, and to my overall health. I have always loved water, so now it is my primary drink to have whenever I am thirsty or with my meals.

You can have fun with water, it does not have to be plain. Assorted natural flavors can make it interesting. Of course, there is the traditional lemon or lime. But you can try fresh strawberry, mint and cucumber, or fresh strawberries and kiwi. Mix it up. Have fun! If you have a juicer, make your own fresh juices without the added sugars and preservatives. But keep in mind juiced fruits are different from whole fruits. The sugar content in juiced fruit is higher than the sugar content in whole fruit.

Now that we have gotten something to snack on while waiting for our meals, we can now dig into those... meals.

Breakfast, lunch, and dinner was the eating schedule we were on, at least most of us. And we have learned that breakfast is the most important meal of the day. Breakfast being the first meal was the heaviest. I remember breakfast tables filled with food. You would have your choice of meats, ham, sausage, or bacon. Eggs, grits, pancakes, and toast. So, from childhood on, this was how breakfast should be. However, being a single mom of 2, working a full-time job, I could not always prepare that grand feast. So, off to McDonalds for the unhealthiest healthy breakfast. And after work, I would prepare meals like spaghetti, lamb chops with rice and vegetables, pasta salad, and things of that nature. (I would not prepare these meals all at once, these dishes were separate meals). Most would think those were pretty "good" meals... not really. I was canceling out the little "good" I was doing at dinner, with breakfast. And I could have prepared the dinners healthier. For example, when making the spaghetti, I should have used zucchini or squash noodles instead of regular pasta noodles since I could not make my own fresh pasta. Or instead of using spaghetti sauce bought in the store which has a lot of sugar in it, make my own sauce. Meat did not have to be in every meal, and it should not be the largest of the portions of food on the plate. A technique I used on myself and my family, was alternating meat with another fruit or vegetable, like mushrooms or jackfruit, one meal a week. Or sometimes I would just omit the meat altogether. Instead of canned or frozen vegetables, use fresh vegetables as much as possible. Before changing my lifestyle, I thought cooking with fresh ingredients would take too long. It does take a little longer, but not too long, and the health benefits are worth the time.

It was easy to alter the dinner ingredients, but breakfast was more of a challenge. As you already know, getting up most mornings was getting harder to do, especially on time. So, preparing a meal in the morning was not an option. The thought that breakfast had to be this massive spread, kept me believing there was just no time to cook in the mornings. I did not really care for breakfast, but it is not just me I am concerned about. There are other passengers on this ride that need nourishment in the mornings. We would stop for the horrible dollar breakfast menu most mornings, but now I know better.

My family likes oatmeal and cereal (later, I found out that most cereals are unhealthy) with almond milk. Sometimes with fresh fruits, granola, or nuts. I will just have a cup of plain, regular coffee. No cream no sugar. If you must eat in the morning, you can have vegetable broth, or toast with a healthy replacement for butter. Avocado toast is a popular thing now, I do not eat it, but my family loves avocado. Eggs scrambled with fresh spinach, garlic, and tomatoes is tasty. Melons are the best in the morning if you really want to lose weight (watermelon, honeydew melon, cantaloupe, etc.). And seeds. Like pumpkin and chia seeds. Breakfast should not be a heavy meal, but should energize you until your next meal, and to cleanse out any remaining particles from last night's meal. (If you need something in between meals, drink water and do not forget about the almonds!). Here come the, "...but I get hungry in between meals, water won't help." We have already touched on the topic of excuses and how they offer no help. Your mental strength comes into play at this point. Time to be your own parent's voice in your head. Wanting to stop doing something just because you can, does not mean you should.

Seasoning is important to those tastebuds. Most of us think that if we have salt and pepper, that is all the seasoning that we need for adequate tasting food The problem with that is, we tend to overcompensate with salt to get more flavor. There is a vast variety of herbs and spices out there that can bring life to your food that will allow you to ease up off the salt.

Experimenting with different herbs and spices is the only way to find out what YOUR tastebuds enjoy. Try experimenting on a day you do not have work or go to school. Just in case you need time to produce a second plan. Start with a small meal, at lunchtime. Research recipes that you may have liked at a restaurant. They usually have a plethora of herbs and spices you do not use at home every day. Maybe cook something you have not cooked before, once or twice a month. After a while, you will have a cabinet of new herbs and spices you did not know existed! With more seasoning, you will need less salt... goals!

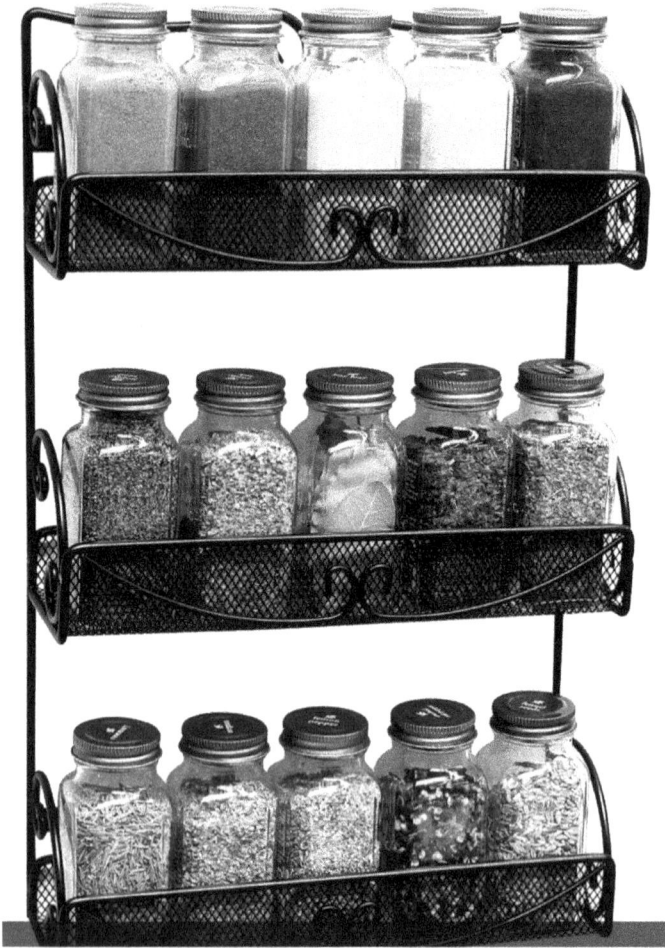

# EXERCISE

You can eat healthy all you want, but the weight will not move if you do not move. You must work out. You must burn calories. Science says that objects in motion remain in motion. Guess what happens to objects that do not remain in motion? You become a couch weight.

I began with something simple, because let us face it, we get lazy over the years. The same routine got comfortable. And it seemed the more I had on my plate, the more I am looking forward to not having to do anything. The first chance I get to do absolutely nothing I am going to take that opportunity. Now I need to find a way to get some extra movement incorporated into my day. So, I began with a leisure walk, nothing too fast, about a quarter of a mile walk around the block. I started off with 10 pushups, 10 sit-ups, and 20 burpees. For someone five foot three and a half inches at about 200 pounds, that was a lot of work. But I kept at it for a few weeks. At about six weeks in is when I realized my workout is getting easier. So now I up my walking distance to a half a mile and increased my speed. I also doubled my sit-ups, push-ups, and burpees. It was about three weeks before I started feeling anxious about not seeing any results from my routine. I am less sluggish, and moving better, but I still look like a blob, you cannot tell where my top ends, and bottom begins. What... is...the problem? The problem is my calorie intake was higher than the calories I was burning. I needed to add some oomph to my workout. It took some time to produce a solution, so I kept my current workout while researching and thinking of a new plan.

One day a thought came to mind. In my younger years, after I had my second child, I felt stiff in certain parts of my body. I had heard about yoga, so I tried it, and it worked great. It also toned my body, without toning being a concern at the time. So, I figured why not try yoga? While sifting through the many online yoga videos, something called Vinyasa yoga popped up. This form of yoga focuses on keeping you moving so you burn calories. Yoga helps stretch out those stiff areas, reduces stress, and increases energy. I made a schedule: Monday cardio, Tuesday yoga, Wednesday cardio, Thursday abs (tired of the blobby looking stomach), Friday cardio. Each workout lasted 20-30 minutes (accept the ab workout, that was only 10 minutes). You can say I slack on ab time, but it works for me. Of course, these are just a couple of activities. There are several others I later found to be effective.

As we get older, our bodies stiffen due to not using certain joints and muscles regularly. Yoga is great for stretching those areas, without having to go through a strenuous workout. It strengthens and tones muscles, while increasing blood flow. My favorite benefit of yoga is the reduction of stress. I would highly suggest yoga to a person with an office job, or someone who sits for lengthy periods of time.

Most people believe cardio means running. Running is one cardio choice, but it is not the only way, and certainly not the best choice. Cardio is for getting the heart pumping, and to increase your body temperature. This is to strengthen your heart and other muscles, and to burn calories.

My favorite cardio workout is swimming. Nothing gets your heart pumping with ease like swimming. You can work out every muscle in the body while getting your heart pumping. The refreshing feel of the water makes me forget I am exercising. And swimming is always fun for me.

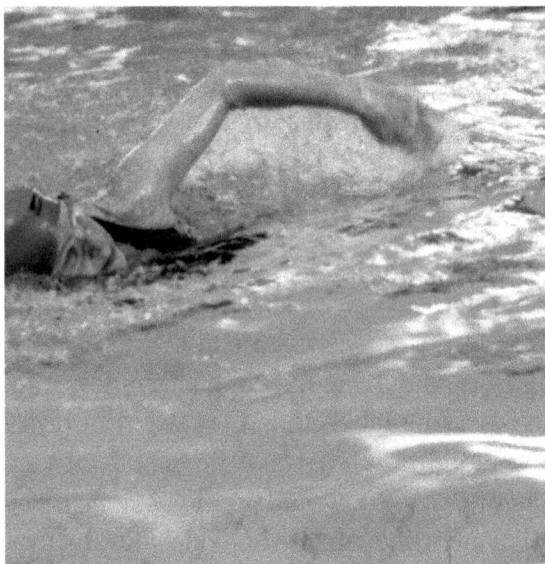

When I cannot get to the pool, walking is my go-to cardio. I take a brisk walk around my neighborhood. When I first started this routine, I did not walk as fast or as far. As time went on, I increased my speed and distance, still not exceeding 30 minutes time. I originally started walking a quarter of a mile. Then I upped it to a half a mile, to a mile. Now I am at a mile and a half.

Of course, you have cycling, burpees, and skating as some other methods you can use for cardio workouts. It is understandable if you live in an area where some of these options are not available year-round, or even available at all. You may have to join a gym, or get creative (run in place, jumping jacks, or jump rope).

Surely the cardio and yoga workouts will touch on the ab and core muscles. However, for defined results, and more strength, there needs to be laser-like focus on the ab area. The ab and core muscles can be tricky to properly strengthen. If you do not work all the muscles in diverse ways, you will not be happy with the outcome.

Sit-ups and crunches are good at working the upper abdominal muscles. There are side and lower abs (internal and external obliques) that also need attention. I like planks for those internal obliques, and leg swings for those external obliques. Planks and palates swimming also help get to those hard-to-reach muscles.

You may look at your gut and think you may have to do more... a lot more. In a way that is true. But do not burn yourself out! Start off slow, just a few repetitions at a time. Besides, if you do too much at once, all will be for not. You will work your butt off, but you will not see any difference. Space your ab workouts so your muscles rest in between workouts. As you can see in my routine, ab day is once a week. You will be surprised to find that a lot of the gut we think is fat, is gas and water retention.

# 29 BEGINNER YOGA POSES

**MOUNTAIN POSE**
Sanskrit Name: Tadasana

**PALM TREE POSE**
(Upward Salute)
Sanskrit Name: Urdhva Hastasana

**STANDING FORWARD BEND (Fold)**
Sanskrit Name: Uttanasan

**HALF STANDING FORWARD BEND**
Sanskrit Name: Ardha Uttanasana

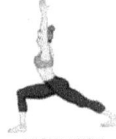

**HIGH LUNGE**
Sanskrit Name:
Utthita Ashwa Sanchalanasana

**CHAIR POSE**
Sanskrit Name: Utkatasana

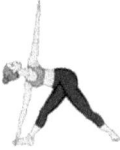

**TRIANGLE POSE**
Sanskrit Name: Trikonasana

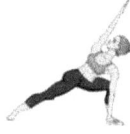

**EXTENDED SIDE ANGLE POSE**
Sanskrit Name:
Utthita Parsvakonasana

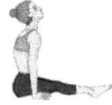

**STAFF POSE**
Sanskrit Name: Dandasana

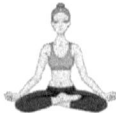

**EASY POSE**
Sanskrit Name: Sukhasana

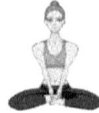

**BOUND ANKLE / COBBLER'S POSE**
Sanskrit Name: Baddha Konasana

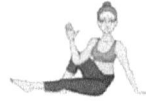

**HALF LORD OF THE FISHES POSE**
Sanskrit Name:
Ardha Matsyendrasana

**TABLE POSE (Table Top Pose)**
Sanskrit Name: Bharmanasana

**CAT POSE**
Sanskrit Name: Marjariasana

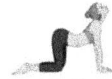

**COW POSE**
Sanskrit Name: Bitilasana

**BALANCING TABLE POSE
(Balancing Table Top Pose)**
Sanskrit Name:
Dandayamana Bharmanasana

**REVERSE TABLE TOP POSE**
Sanskrit Name:
Ardha Purvottanasana

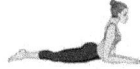

**SPHINX POSE**
Sanskrit Name:
Salamba Bhujangasana

**COBRA POSE**
Sanskrit Name: Bhujangasana

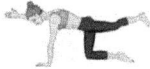

**BIG TOE POSE**
Sanskrit Name: Padangusthasana

**CHILD'S POSE**
Sanskrit Name: Balasana

**ONE-LEGGED BOAT POSE**
Sanskrit Name:
Ekapada Navasana

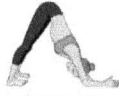

**DOLPHIN POSE**
Sanskrit Name: Catur Svanasana

**BRIDGE POSE**
Sanskrit Name:
Sethu Bandha Sarvangasana

**GARLAND POSE
(Frog Squat Pose)**
Sanskrit Name: Malasana

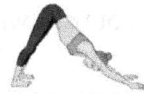

**DOWNWARD-FACING DOG POSE**
Sanskrit Name:
Adho Mukha Svanasana

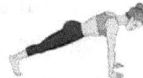

**PLANK POSE**
Sanskrit Name: Kumbhakasana

**CHATURANGA**
Sanskrit Name:
Chaturanga Dandasana

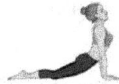

**UPWARD-FACING DOG**
Sanskrit Name:
Urdhva Mukha Svanasana

Make note, your diet also affects your results. Overeating meat, bread, salt, and processed sugar help contribute to that famous tire around our waists. So, if you love those things, it is time for some self-discipline, also known as self-love. Cut those things down or completely out if you can. At least until you reach your goal. However, I would not suggest bringing processed sugar back into your diet.

Do not misunderstand, there were times, in the beginning of my journey when I would skip a workout day. Sometimes I would go a whole week or longer without working out. But after about six weeks, things changed. I no longer wanted to miss any of my workouts. If I missed any days, I would feel guilty. I felt like I was missing something. During the times I took longer breaks I noticed that it was harder to back on track. So, breaks in between workouts narrowed. I no longer craved sweets and processed foods the way I did before. My body craved healthier foods and had no desire for the opposite. It no longer felt like an undesirable chore to eat healthy and workout.

Now I am starting to notice the pounds melt like butter... 198lbs... 176lbs... The pounds shredded quickly, until I got down to the last 20 pounds I wanted to lose. That seemed like it took forever to get rid of, but I did. I got the reward for my work with a glance in the full-body mirror for sticking to my plan. The journey was arduous however, I made it through.

# FASTING

In the last book I omitted this topic because it was controversial, and I was still learning about my own experiences with the tool. I should have still at least mentioned it since it was a huge factor in my weight loss. Conversations I had with others reveal that a lot of people are not aware of the positive effects of fasting. Intermitted fasting is safest for beginners to get a feel for how the body and mind reacts to fasting. Tracking when and what you eat keeps you aware of your diet intake. And fasting is a form of cleaning and regenerating your body. Excreting old dead cells and creating new youthful cells, fasting brings youthfulness back to the body.

During my journey, 3 months into it, I began intermitted fasting. In the morning (7 AM), I would have nothing but plain tea. Between 11-11:30 AM I would eat my meal for the day and have small snacks until 7 PM. For the rest of the evening until bedtime I would have nothing but plain tea and water. I continued this routine for a few weeks until I was able to challenge myself to an extended fast of 36 hours once a week. There were times when I felt so good after my 36 hours of fasting that I would continue to fast for 72 hours. So far, the longest fast have been on was 96 hours. I continued to workout during the times I fasted and felt fine. I felt great!

The most important thing to remember when fasting is nourishment before and after. Of the two the biggest is after the fast. Diving right back into the regular diet routine can cause harm to your body. Your digestive system must be prepared to get back to its regular flow and you want the most bang for your buck when you start putting food back into your body. What I mean is, you do not want empty foods going into the empty vessel. You want foods that are going to help your body run at its maximum ability. Foods that nourish yet help aid in weight loss. One example of a break fast (breakfast) is warmed bone broth, sliced cucumbers, and pumpkin seeds. You have some fats and protein by having the broth. The cucumbers provide vitamin K, magnesium, potassium, fiber (with the skin on) and aids in weight loss. Pumpkin seeds give you more of the protein and fats that you get from beef broth but also has fiber, zinc, and iron. When you eat foods that give the body something to use as fuel, you will eat less. Compared to when you feed your body empty foods you keep looking for something to eat more often than you should.

Now that you have cleansed your body of the toxins that harm your body, you can focus on foods that help energize your body. I know we are all used to the notion of we need to eat to survive. We do need to eat but we also need to fast because all foods, in some way, are toxic to the body. That is a topic for another book another time.

# RECAP

Recognizing there is a problem with oneself is one of the hardest things to do. We go through denial, and we make excuses. You have never, nor will you ever see an excuse resolve a problem. Thought, plan, and action should replace denial, excuse, and procrastination. Just sitting down, writing out a plan is a start. It does not have to be perfect at first. There is always room for adjustment along the way. Writing out your plan gets your mind prepared for the action. Mental preparation helps to get the rest of body to cooperate. The mind and body need to coordinate for best results. No room for negative thinking. Nothing but positivity from now on.

The body needs routine, and stability helps. It is important to have a place to rest, exercise, and prepare your meals. The body has its own clock. Keeping on routine keeps the body running at its maximum performance.

If you must snack, snack clean, no processed foods and processed sugars. Processed foods have no nutritional value, so if you are feeding your body these foods, you are starving your body at the same time. Drink plenty of water because hydration helps the system with cleansing. Toxins in the body contribute to poor health.

Exercise does not have to be grueling, find what pushes you, yet makes you comfortable while having fun. Start off slow, then gradually increase the reps and difficulty of your workout. If you isolate the parts of the body, you work out, i.e., abdominal muscles or legs, make sure you space out the days. You want to make sure you see results promptly. Please keep in mind that everyone is different. You and your friend may start working out at the same time, but one may show results quicker than the other. In discouraging times do not give up! Stick to the plan and you will get what you are looking for.

Fasting is huge in weight loss and maintenance. It helps rid the body of toxins and rejuvenate cells that creates a youthful look and feel for the body. It does take willpower and accountability to fast. However, it can be dangerous when done incorrectly. Be sure to nourish properly and stay hydrated. After fasting becomes routine, it will be easier to do. Once you have reached your desired weight, you can space out the fasting times. At this point your eating should be cleaner and you will not need to fast as often as when you first began your journey.

A lot of times we will make excuses for ourselves. You might say you are too tired. There will be some aches and pains that bother you. Or you do not have the time. Have you ever heard the saying, "I'm sick and tired of being sick and tired"? When you are at your most fed-up moment of being overweight. When you are through the being fatigued and sickly. When you have had it with all the doctor's visits. When you are, "sick and tired of being sick and tired," you will want to change. And when you want to change, nothing and no one can stop you.

# RECIPES

## COWBOY CAVIAR

Ingredients

*For the vinaigrette:*

>2 tablespoons olive oil
>Finely grated zest of 1 medium lime
>Juice of 1 medium lime
>1 teaspoon kosher salt
>1 teaspoon ground cumin
>1/4 teaspoon chili powder
>1/4 teaspoon dried oregano
>1/4 teaspoon freshly ground black pepper

*For the cowboy caviar:*

>1 (15-ounce) can black-eyed peas, drained and rinsed
>1 (15-ounce) can black beans, drained and rinsed
>3 cloves garlic, minced
>2 medium Roma or plum tomatoes, seeded and diced
>1 medium orange bell pepper, seeded and diced small

1 medium green bell pepper, seeded and diced small

1 medium jalapeño pepper, seeded and minced

1/4 medium red onion, small dice

1 cup fresh or thawed frozen corn kernels

Chopped fresh cilantro

**Make the vinaigrette:** Place all the ingredients in a large bowl and whisk until well-combined.

Add the black-eyed peas, black beans, garlic, tomatoes, bell pepper, jalapeño, red onion, and corn to the bowl of dressing and toss until well-coated. Refrigerate for at least 1 hour, then toss again and garnish with cilantro. Serve with tortilla chips, on a salad, or in a tortilla.

## MAKES

about 5 1/2 cups; serves 8 to 12 as an appetizer

## Roasted Asparagus

### Ingredients

1- and 1/2-pounds asparagus, woody ends removed

2 tablespoons avocado oil

1 tablespoon unsalted butter, melted

1/2 teaspoon EACH: fine sea salt, dried Italian seasoning

1/4 teaspoon EACH: garlic powder, freshly cracked pepper

1/3 cup Panko (or breadcrumbs - Note 1)

1/3 cup + 2 tablespoons freshly grated Parmesan cheese, separated

### Instructions

Preheat the oven to 425 degrees F. Grab your largest baking sheet (I recommend a 15×21-inch sheet pan).

Wash under cool water and dry COMPLETELY (do this quickly, by rolling the spears in between two kitchen towels). Snap off the woody ends from each asparagus spear.

Place the asparagus spears directly on your large sheet pan. Drizzle over the olive oil and melted butter. Add the salt, Italian seasoning, garlic powder, and pepper. Toss until the spears are well coated. They need to have enough oil + butter so the panko & parmesan will stick; pour an added tablespoon of oil IF needed (if you have more than 1.5 pounds asparagus)

Finally, sprinkle on top the Panko and 1/3 cup Parmesan cheese (I like grating it with a micro plane/zester for the perfect texture). Again, toss gently to ensure the panko and parmesan coats all the spears.

Spread the asparagus into one even layer ensuring they are not overlapping (otherwise you would be steaming instead of roasting the asparagus; separate to 2 sheet pans as needed). Some of the panko/parmesan will fall to the tray and that is fine. Sprinkle more of the mixture on the spears if needed.

Bake 7-11 minutes or until spears are lightly browned, tender, and the Parmesan cheese is melted. (May vary depending on actual oven temperature and size of spears). Remove from the oven and sprinkle the remaining 2 tablespoons Parmesan cheese on the hot asparagus. I like to grab some of the toasted Panko from the tray and add it on top of the bowl or platter of spears!

Enjoy at once while hot

# ROASTED KALE CHIPS

## Ingredients

1 bunch kale about 6 cups, loosely packed
1 TBS avocado oil
¼ tsp sea salt (do not over salt!)

## Instructions

Preheat oven to 325 degrees F.
Lightly grease a large baking sheet, set aside.
Remove the leafy green part of the kale from the tough stalk, and tear into smaller pieces.
Place kale leaves into a large mixing bowl.
Add 1 TBS avocado oil to the kale and massage with your hands until every single piece has oil. (This step is especially important for the sea salt to stick).
If necessary, add more avocado oil 1 tsp at a time until the oil is all over.
Sprinkle the salt over the oil-coated kale chips.
Toss the mixture carefully with tongs to evenly distribute the oil and salt on the kale chips. (careful to not over handle).
Bake for 10-15 minutes or until the kale is crispy and just begins to brown. Stir halfway through.
Once brown and crispy, let cool completely on the baking sheet.

Remove cooled kale chips from the baking sheet and eat or put in a container with a loosely fitting lid to store.

# SPAGHETTI SAUCE

## Ingredients

6 garlic cloves minced
1 TBSP avocado oil
28 oz crushed tomatoes
28 oz diced tomatoes
1/2 tsp kosher salt
1/2 tsp dried oregano
1/2 tsp dried parsley
1/2 tsp dried basil
1/8 tsp crushed red pepper flakes optional
pepper to taste

## Instructions

Heat the avocado oil in a large sauce pan over medium heat. Add the garlic and sauté just until it becomes fragrant, about 30 seconds.

Add in the crushed and diced tomatoes. Stir in the salt, oregano, parsley, basil, and crushed red pepper flakes. Add pepper to taste.

Bring the sauce to a simmer and cook on low for about 15 minutes or until the sauce is thickens, stirring intermittently.

# AVOCADO TOAST

## Ingredients

1 slice of bread
½ ripe avocado
Pinch of salt
Pinch of fresh ground black pepper
Squeeze of lime juice

## Instructions

Toast your slice of bread until golden and firm.Remove the pit from your avocado. Use a big spoon to scoop out the flesh. Put it in a bowl and mash it up with a fork until it is as smooth as you like it. Mix in lime juice, black pepper, and a pinch of salt (about ⅛ teaspoon) and add more to taste, if desired.

Spread avocado on top of your toast.

# Veggie Burgers

## Ingredients

15 oz cooked black beans
3/4 cup of cooked wild rice
17 oz mushrooms
Rice cooked in chicken broth/bouillon
½ cup flour
½ cup cornstarch
Avocado oil
1 tsp Black pepper
½ tbsp Cumin
½ tbsp Rosemary
1tsp Thyme
1 tsp Liquid smoke
Salt to taste

## Instructions

In a large mixing bowl, combine all ingredients except the flour and cornstarch, mix those in a separate bowl together. The flour and cornstarch mix is to be slowly added to the other mixture. The caution is to avoid dry patties while still keeping the binding of your patty. Add your mushroom and bean mix to a blender or food processor with half of the flour and cornstarch mix. Continue blending for approximately 5 minutes or until all ingredients are well blended. The consistency should be similar to raw ground beef. If the mix is too wet, continue to slowly add more flour to the mix. Once you have the desired consistency, create balls in the size of patty you would like and set them aside. In your favorite frying pan, cover the bottom of the pan with enough oil to coat the pan, add a little extra so theres some oil left in the pan after the initial submergence of the patty so your patties do not stick to the bottom of the pan. Fry each side about 3 minutes each. Remove from the pan and serve on your favorite bun. I enjoy a brioche bun, mustard, barbecue sauce (JJBBBQ), fresh red onions, tomatoes, spinach, and cucumbers.


## Lions Mane Gumbo


Ingredients

1 tbsp oil
1 onion diced
1 green bell pepper, diced
3 large celery stalks, diced
2 cloves garlic, minced
6 cups broth (chicken or vegetable)
14 oz can tomatoes, diced
½ cup okra, diced
2 small zucchini, diced
½ pound lions mane mushrooms (bite size pieces)
1 tsp gumbo filé
1 tsp salt
¼ tbsp ground black pepper
2 tbsp hot sauce

2 tsp cornstarch dissolved in ½ cup cold water
Cooked rice

## Instructions

In a soup pot, sauté the onion, garlic and mushrooms over a low-moderate heat. Add the bell pepper and celery and cook a few more minutes. Add the seasonings, tomato and zucchini and partially cover. Simmer for about 25 minutes. If you prefer a thicker stew, add the cornstarch and return the stew to a moderate heat for a few minutes. Adjust salt and pepper. Serve over a fluffy cooked rice.

## Lo Mein

### Ingredients

3 tbsp oyster sauce
1tsp sesame oil
1 tbsp soy sauce
¼ cup chicken broth
1 tbsp cornstarch
3 tbsp avocado oil
2 tsp garlic, minced
1 ½ tbsp ginger, thinly sliced
1 pound mushrooms (your choice)(I like oyster
mushrooms for this dish)(chicken is an option too!)
3 cups lo mein noodles (chow mein, egg, or pancit,
noodles), cooked fresh
¼ pound baby bok choy, bottoms removed
3 spring onions, sliced 1 ½ inch

### Instructions

Sauce: In a small bowl, stir together the oyster sauce,
sesame oil, soy sauce, chicken broth, and cornstarch.

Lo Mein dish
Heat a wok or large skillet over high heat and add
cooking oil. Once you see wisps of white smoke, add the

garlic and ginger. Stir while cooking until the ginger and garlic are light brown and fragrant, about 20 seconds.
Add in mushrooms, continue cooking and stirring for approximately 1 minute.
Stir in the noodles and bok choy. Continue cooking, stirring, and tossing, until the bok choy starts to soften and turn bright green, approximately 1 minute.
Stir in the sauce; allow the sauce to coat all the ingredients, and simmer for approximately 1 minute.
Continue cooking, stirring and tossing until your protein (mushrooms) are thoroughly cooked through, and the sauce starts to bubble, approximately 1 minute.
Top with spring onions.
Serve hot.

I have altered all recipes to fit my taste. You can do the same!

Deidra Jones

Copyright © 2025 Deidra Jones

www.ingramcontent.com/pod-product-compliance
Lightning Source LLC
Chambersburg PA
CBHW052106270326
41931CB00012B/2910